How To Eat Healthy and Feel Awesome

308 Great Tips To Nutrition And Healthy Eating

ADAM COLTON

Published by BizMove
www.bizmove.com

Copyright © 2017 Liraz Publishing

All rights reserved.

ISBN: 1979495408
ISBN- 978-1979495400

308 Great Tips To Nutrition And Healthy Eating

So you have decided that it is time to eat healthy. The only thing you know is that it's hard to change something that you have been doing all your life. The tips that you will find in this book will help you lead a nutritious life and to keep with it.

1. Try to avoid fad diets. Many of these are not tailored to fit everybody's different nutritional and health-related needs, so doing some of these without consulting a physician can be dangerous. many leave out important daily nutrients that your body needs. Stick to things like lean meats, watching your fats, cholesterol and sugars,and eating healthy produce with a lot of water.

2. Calcium is a beneficial mineral that should be a part of a healthy diet. Calcium is involved in teeth and bone structure. It also helps in blood clotting, nerve function, muscle contraction, and blood vessel contraction. Calcium helps prevent many diseases such as osteoporosis, hypertension, diabetes, colon cancer, high cholesterol, and obesity.

3. Put a lot of fiber in your diet. Foods with a lot of fiber in them such as nuts and whole-grains are great. Because the fiber takes a long time to break

down in the body, you feel full for longer than with other foods. This way you won't have cravings for junk food as often.

4. Milk is the best form of liquid protein you can give you body. Packed full of protein, vitamin D and other important nutrients, milk is a natural, affordable drink, that everyone should take advantage of. Instead of using protein shakes to bulk up, consider drinking two or three glasses of milk every day, instead.

5. Nutrition is key to any successful exercise routine, so be sure not to let your body run out of fuel. If you are going to exercise for more than 90 minutes, you will need to replenish your store of energy. Eat 50 to 60 grams of carbohydrates for each hour you plan to exercise.

6. As you grocery shop, make sure your children are involved in the process. Let them choose which fruits and vegetables they want to eat. Doing this can also entice children to try out new foods, especially those with bright colors.

7. A great nutrition tip is to start incorporating flax seed into your diet. Flax seed is an amazing source of essential fatty acids and it's very easy to add to food. You can sprinkle a bit of flax seed in your

protein shake, or you can put a little bit in your salad.

8. If you are a vegetarian, make sure your nutrition choices are well-rounded. While many omnivores miss essential vitamins in their diet, it's easier to recover lost minerals. That said, it's easy to keep on top of a vegetarian diet. If you find yourself hitting roadblocks, consider seeing a nutritionist.

9. Give canned salmon a try if you want a different taste sensation. It is full of vitamins and minerals your body needs and is low fat. Try varying meals as much as you can to enjoy your daily diet plan.

10.   Many dieticians recommend replacing red meats in your diet with fish. If you had tried fish once or twice in the past but really don't see it as something that you could ever eat on a daily basis, remember that there are dozens of different types of fish. Whether you opt for mackerel, mullet, snapper, sardines, or flounder, each kind has its own distinctive flavor and texture. Just because you did not like or two kinds does not mean you will not like any of them.

11.   Tape your goal to your bath room mirror, to your refrigerator, your computer monitor, and even your television remote. Whenever you look in the

mirror, you will be reminded of how you are bettering your life. When you go to open the refrigerator, it will remind you that you need to eat healthy.

12.   If you're pregnant, make sure you're getting enough iron in your diet. For a normal adult woman you should be taking in 18mg a day of iron, but during pregnancy this should be upped to 27mg a day. The baby needs a lot of iron to develop and if you don't have enough it can cause anemia which can cause problems for you and the baby.

13.   Try to shop smart when buying whole grain foods. You can't depend on the color of a food to determine its grain content. For example, a product called '100% wheat', 'multi-grain', 'cracked wheat' or 'stone-ground' is not a guarantee that it is 100% whole grain. Always go over the list of ingredients and the table of nutritional values.

14.   Make sure to reward each of your small victories with friends and family. If you reward yourself with a meal or food make sure the reward is healthy. You don't want to keep rewarding yourself with bad food as this will return you to some of your old bad habits.

15.   It is not all about counting points or counting calories. It is all about controlling your insulin levels and eating food that is good for you. If you follow a diet of nutrient-dense food, you are sure to have much more success in maintaining a healthy weight.

16.   To get kids to eat a more nutritious diet, sometimes you have to make compromises. Because children have not fully developed their taste buds, they tend to be picky eaters. To get them to try something new, combine it with something they already love. The most obvious example of this tactic is to combine vegetables with cheese.

17.   A good nutrition tip for health conscious people is to keep their annual and semi-annual checkups. This includes doctors exams as well as dentist exams too. Woman should also remember to get breast exams after the age of 30 and they should also give themselves breast self-examinations once a month.

18.   Do not make the mistake of avoiding fat entirely. Some fat is necessary to provide a feeling of fullness and help your body function properly, but try to stick to healthier fats rather than the partially hydrogenated version found in most packaged snack food. A little fat with a meal causes carbohydrates to digest more slowly for a lower rise

in blood sugar, resulting in more constant energy and less hunger later.

19.   Even artificial sweeteners can raise your blood sugar and insulin levels in much the same way as sugar. Although they may be lower in calories, they are not necessarily any more healthy. Instead change on how much you depend on sweet things. Start by cutting your sugars in half and work you way to not needing them at all.

20.   When considering your child's nutrition, it is important to keep them involved throughout the whole process. This will excite the child because of the sense of importance they will feel. Bring them to the store with you and have them help you pick out foods that they like and that are healthy. Be sure to not give into purchasing everything that the child desires. When back home, have them help you with the meal preparation.

21.   Omega 3 fatty acids are a key part of a nutritionally balanced diet. They help your heart, organs and blood remain healthy and are increasingly accepted by the medical community as a great way to stay healthy. You can find Omega 3 fatty acids in fish products or by taking a pill.

22.   A great nutrition tip is to overcome emotional eating. A lot of people tend to eat food as a way of coping with stress. This is known as emotional eating it can lead to obesity and low self-esteem. By overcoming emotional eating, you'll be much healthier and in a better place.

23.   Moderate your alcohol intake. Sugary calories, which are abundant in alcoholic drinks, are easily converted to fat stored in your body. Also, when there is alcohol in your body, it causes your liver to work overtime to process it and burn fat. Excess alcohol intake can cause many threatening health conditions.

24.   Help your child to become interested in new foods by describing the texture, rather than the taste. They may be interested by your description of its texture and then be willing to try eating it.

25.   Nutrition during pregnancy has special requirements to ensure that your baby is as healthy as possible. Focusing on iron-rich foods will make sure that your developing baby will have an adequate oxygen supply during development. Iron-rich foods can also help prevent premature delivery. Good sources of iron include lean meat, chicken and fish.

26.   Always carry healthy snacks around with you. That is a good idea because most of the time people cheat on diets because healthier options are not available to them at the time. Keeping nuts, dried fruits, sugar free candy and sliced vegetables around will satisfy any cravings you get.

27.   Add green tea to your diet. Green tea contains polyphenols, which are powerful antioxidants. It has anti-inflammatory properties that can protect the skin and benefit its overall health. Drinking green tea can help to reduce the damage from sunburn, in turn reducing the risk of skin cancer. Try to drink two cups of green tea per day.

28.   Plan your consumption of fruit. Fruit is quite beneficial in a diet but if you want to control your insulin levels better, only eat it after doing physical exercise. It may be fine for some people to eat it for breakfast but if you feel as if you are having trouble with your insulin levels, only consume after physical exertion.

29.   Take two 300-milligram capsules of Omega-3 supplements twice a day, about 30 minutes prior to lunch and dinner. The hormone cholecystokinin is released which reduces your appetite. Another benefit of Omega-3 is its effective anti-inflammatory benefits and the reduction of high

triglycerides, which are a risk factor for heart disease.

30.   Do not discount fiber in your nutrition goals. Fiber comes from sources like, grains, beans, fresh fruits, vegetables, and various other sources. Increasing your fiber during meals will extend your feelings of fullness and help your body in its efforts to remove waste. Getting rid of much of the waste that can be forgotten in your system will allow your body to function more normally.

31.   When dining out, you should choose to eat meats that are not breaded or fried. These foods will be loaded with grease and fats. A healthier alternative is to choose meats that are grilled, broiled or baked. Just about any meat can be cooked in the healthier way and it will taste much better too.

32.   It is important to incorporate at least 5 servings of fruits and vegetables into your diet every day. Fruits and vegetables are very healthy and help your body to get the fibers, antioxidants and vitamins that it needs. They also help fill up your stomach fast so you are able to feel full longer. Fruits and vegetables are low in calories so they help to keep your calorie count low.

33. If you're having a treat, try and minimize the damage by making it diet-friendly. Pizza should be balanced, and your toppings might have a ratio of a quarter meat to two-thirds vegetables to represent your newly varied diet. This will help you cut back on calories and fat, even with rewards.

34. Vitamin D is an important part of a healthy diet. It assists in bone and teeth formation by maintaining calcium and phosphorous levels in the body. Vitamin D also helps in immune function and cell growth. Lowering cancer risk is yet another benefit of vitamin D.

35. Put a lot of fiber in your diet. Foods with a lot of fiber in them such as nuts and whole-grains are great. Because the fiber takes a long time to break down in the body, you feel full for longer than with other foods. This way you won't have cravings for junk food as often.

36. One of the most important, yet difficult, ways to achieve proper nutrition is to break any addiction to junk foods and sweets. Long-standing unhealthy eating habits accustom someone to the ease and deliciousness of junk food. You can want to have these unhealthy foods long after you stopped eating them. Realize when you are craving bad foods and eat something good for you!

37.   Making sure that you're giving your body the proper nutrition that it needs can be hard at times. Taking a daily multivitamin can help ensure that some of your nutritional needs are always met. Many daily multivitamins provide a full day's worth of several vitamins and minerals that your body needs in one small pill.

38.   When eating out, ask your server for his or her recommendations. Restaurants often specifically train their servers to be very familiar with the menu. The next time you find yourself eating out, do not be afraid to question the staff. They will likely be able to point out to you, the healthiest choices on the menu.

39.   When considering your nutrition, be sure to watch out for foods that may appear healthy but end up being quite the opposite. There can be a lot of hidden fat and sodium in otherwise healthy looking snacks. Smoothies can end up having a lot of fat calories and sugar depending on the ingredients used. Energy bars can be a hidden source of a large amount of calories. Fat free foods can contain the same amount of calories as regular versions.

40.   Next time you want a snack, grab a handful of blueberries. Blueberries are packed with nutrients that are vital to your body. They provide a high level of vitamin C. They also contain antioxidant properties that protect your cell tissue from being damaged by free radicals. Blueberries may also have potential benefits in the fight against cancer.

41.   Read and understand the labels on the food you buy. The nutrition labels list the serving size, the calories, the fat, the sodium, the cholesterol, the carbohydrate, the protein and the vitamin content of each serving. Using this information you can calculate how much you have to eat from each type of food.

42.   Rice is one of the most convenient foods that you can have, as it is very easy to make and goes with a wide variety of foods. Instead of white rice, choose brown rice, as it is healthier for your body and contains a lower level of fat content upon consumption.

43.   When you are developing an eating plan, make sure that you do not set up any meals after 7 p.m. This will give your body the chance to digest at the end of the night and improve the way that you feel in the morning. Eat dinner at 6, and do not consume anything heavy afterwards.

44.   When you go shopping, have a list of planned meals. Going to a store with a specific list will help you not to deviate from the foods you should be eating. This will also make sure that you have all the ingredients on hand to make the right kinds of foods when you're at home instead of ordering take out.

45.   It is important to get enough iron in your diet, because it is used for oxygen transport throughout the body. If you do not get enough, you will suffer from anemia. Good sources of iron include meat, particularly organ meats like liver, dark leafy vegetables such as spinach, and molasses.

46.   Remember to drink lots of water throughout the day. It has many benefits unrelated to diet as well but when you are trying to lose weight it can help to satisfy the psychological need to put something in your mouth and stomach. It will also help to feel more full even when you are not.

47.   Avoid the desire to simultaneously change every aspect in your life. Write down what you want to do, and diligently mark things off as you go. Begin with the things that are impacting your health the most and move on from there.

48.   While nutrition is great and very important for a healthy lifestyle, don't let it become your identity. You eat healthy because it is the best way to live not because you want to be known as the person who eats correctly. Once you let it become an obsession than you have returned to the same problems as you had before.

49.   Looking for an quick and easy way to sneak those eight 8oz of water in that experts recommend you drink each and every day? Drink two full glasses of water with each meal, and carry around a 16os water bottle with you during the day to sip from occasionally.

50.   High fructose corn syrup, sugar, and other forms of carbohydrates are all essentially the same when it comes to nutrition. They might react in a different manner with the body, diffusing sugar faster, but they all carry similar calorie contents and behave like sugars. Starches like bread and pasta provide a large portion of carbohydrates which allows you to store up energy in fat cells.

51.   If you are trying to eat as cheaply as possible, but still want to be healthy, purchase a variety of fortified breakfast cereals. Vitamins and minerals are added so it's as if you're taking a multivitamin.

One box provides you with 4 or 5 meals so the cost per meal is less than one dollar for you.

52.   Soy has been known to be a great addition to any healthy diet. It has been shown to help prevent diseases like heart disease and cancer because of its essential fatty acids, iron, phosphorus, and other nutrients. It is great for eliminating blockages in arteries too. Soy also helps reduce cholesterol levels.

53.   In order to have a healthy body, it is important to eat breakfast every day. It is the most important meal of the day because it improves your cognitive skills and provides the necessary energy needed throughout the day. Studies show that people who eat breakfast, tend to eat less during the day.

54.   An unknown boon to many, studies have shown that red wine is actually a healthy choice. Compared to white wine, red wine has less sugar and more healthy nutrients. Nutritionists believe that drinking one glass of red wine per day may increase your life expectancy. The same idea applies to dark chocolate.

55.   It's often said that processed grains taste much better than whole grains. White flour might be the only option for some recipes. Nonetheless, whole grains are far more healthful in terms of fiber and

nutrition, and you can usually substitute about a quarter whole grain flour in almost any baked goods recipe successfully.

56.   Leeks, garlic and onions are sometimes frowned upon due to their odor. But if you have avoided them, you should reconsider. They provide B and C vitamins and help liver function. Many studies have indicated their properties in deterring cancer. Cooking them in complex dishes, reduces their strong odor.

57.   You want to try and keep a routine with your kid's meal times. Try to serve meals and snacks at roughly the same time every day. Let your child have juice or milk at meal times only, and drink water the rest of the time. If they drink juice and milk all day, they may not have an appetite later.

58.   You might buy ground turkey thinking that it's lower fat, and therefore better for you nutritionally. But you should always read the labels, and ground turkey is no exception. Ground turkey contains both white and dark meat, the latter being high in fat. And ground turkey, though certainly leaner than ground hamburger, is actually higher in fat than ground sirloin.

59.   Save your used drink bottles, fill them with water and freeze them. Having water available to quench your thirst is imperative to good health. Frozen water bottles will likely stay cool all day and an added wellness benefit, is that they are handy to grab to wet down a wipe and cool yourself off on hot days.

60.   A great nutritional tip is to turn off the television so that it won't distract your child when he or she eats. Eating in front of the television can lead to poor eating habits and it makes you unaware of how much you're eating. Get your child to focus on eating instead of watching television.

61.   While nuts are very nutritious, you still need to choose correctly. Raw almonds are a great snack that contain lots of healthy fiber, as well as having a satisfying, tasty crunch.

62.   Enjoy a drink now and again. Countless studies have shown that a drink now and then, whether it be a glass of wine or beer, is actually good for you. A certain amount of alcohol can help to lower the incidence of cardiovascular disease. That being said, you should aim for a low-alcohol version, which is obviously, lower in calories.

63.   Not everyone likes to talk about it, but everybody knows it: Fiber keeps your regular. Meeting your recommended daily allowance of fiber is easier than ever with commercially prepared over-the-counter fiber supplements, not to mention the abundance of fiber found naturally in popular foods like oats, whole grains, lettuce, fresh spinach, and most other vegetables. Getting enough fiber also helps to lower your risk of developing heart disease and certain types of diabetes.

64.   Always try to have sugarless chewing gum on hand since chewing that can help satisfy sweet cravings and general food cravings. When you get hungry, popping a piece of gum in your mouth actually seems to take the food cravings from you right away and you can wait to eat until it is time for your next meal.

65.   For a festive and fun meal that the family will enjoy, make kabobs on the grill or under the broiler. This is great for kids because they can choose the veggies and meat that go on their kabob. Make the colors bright and cheerful so that they will want to make theirs as pretty (and veggie filled) as possible.

66.   A great nutrition tip is to make sure you eat a proper meal before you work out. You'll want something that will digest fast and give you instant

energy. Fruits are good to eat before working out. Avoid food that's high in fat because it'll sit in your stomach.

67.   Nutrition isn't something you just "do." You also have to learn how to do it. That means researching product labels and understanding exactly what it is that you're putting into your body. A lot of the time "fat-free" doesn't mean that it has no fat, it may just be a way to draw a consumer in. Also sugar free or carbohydrate free doesn't necessarily mean that it's lower in calories.

68.   Sometimes it is better to add things to your diet rather than remove them. If you absolutely do not have the willpower to replace all those unhealthy snack foods you eat with fruits and vegetables, eat the fruits and vegetables anyway. Slowly begin to phase the snack foods out when you feel you can.

69.   When you are trying to decide what to have for dinner, remember that you should have equal amounts of vegetable and grains on your plate. You will be able to get full without eating too much of the calorie-ridden grains. This is because a cup of grains has about 200 calories and the veggies have just 50 or so.

70.   Eat healthful foods to keep your whole body fit and healthy. Your skin will glow if you eat plenty of fresh fruits and veggies, whole grains, proteins, and natural oils. Be sure to get plenty of good oils, such as olive oil, sunflower oil and peanut oil to keep your skin, hair, and nails moisturized, flexible and strong.

71.   Eat raw foods. As you get older, your body has a harder time digesting foods, making it less likely that you will be able to extract all the vitamins and nutrients from processed and cooked foods. Raw foods have more nutrients, therefore it's easier for your digestive system to access them.

72.   For best nutrition, be sure to choose fats wisely. Butter was once thought to be the enemy due to the high amount of saturated fat. However, margarine has been found to be high in trans fats, which are unhealthy for the heart. Best would be to limit your fats as much as possible; second best would be one of the "Smart Balance" non-trans-fat type margarine's, and third best would be to use real butter, but very sparingly.

73.   When you are looking for a meal that is easy to make and still gives you a lot of nutrition, try a baked potato. They offer a lot of fiber, and if you

leave off the sour cream and butter, you will have a lower calorie meal with less fat.

74.   Make sure most of your meals or snacks includes some protein, and try to get an adequate amount of healthy fat each day. Both fat and protein will make you feel more satified than if you got the same number of calories from a sugary snack. Additionally, protein is necessary if you're exercising as well as dieting, to ensure that you don't lose too much muscle along with fat.

75.   Eat oatmeal for breakfast. Oatmeal is a great source of fiber, protein and whole grains. It will fill you up, keep you full and help to clean the cholesterol out of your system. Oatmeal can be eaten plain, or with whole fruit added to sweeten it up.

76.   Most people do not eat enough zinc on a daily basis. It is vital for the functioning of many important enzymes in the human body, as well as, being necessary for healthy male reproductive health. It can be found in such foods as wheat, beans, nuts and other seeds. It is better to eat zinc in food rather than using supplements.

77.   If you suspect any nutritional deficiencies, consider going to your doctor to check for

underlying medical conditions. You may have an intolerance or reaction to certain foods, making it difficult to maintain a healthy regimen. Oftentimes, these problems can be masked, or cause nonspecific issues that take some time to work out. Your doctor can help you determine for sure.

78.   Soybeans are practically miraculous in their nutritional value. They contain a moderate amount of carbohydrates, lots of good protein, and just enough fat to help you absorb the good phytochemicals like isoflavones and the omega-3 fatty acids. Eating more protein in the form of soy products will also help you avoid saturated fats and cholesterol.

79.   Fresh whole fruit is a better option than fruit juice. Fruit juice is usually artificially sweetened, while fresh fruit is 100% natural. The amount of sugar in some fruit juices is higher than the amount of sugar in soft drinks. Whole fruit offers crucial vitamins, minerals and fiber which may prevent some chronic diseases, including cardiovascular issues.

80.   If you are searching for a vitamin that helps to reduce depression and sadness, look no further than vitamin B-12. This vitamin is a great addition to your morning arsenal, as it will help to put you in a

good mood so that you will have the motivation to exercise and eat well all day.

81.	Consume whole grains as a regular part of your diet. Whole grains have been proven to reduce your risk of heart disease and diabetes. They have the ability to help you maintain healthy blood sugar levels. Avoid over-processed white bread products and instead, choose whole grains.

82.	A healthy diet will help to boost your immune system. By boosting your body's immune system your body will be able to fight against the impurities that cause skin problems. Just keeping track of what you are putting in your body and making sure that what you put in your body boosts the immune system.

83.	Avoid substituting fruit juices for whole fruits. Whole fruits are fresher and will offer you a higher nutritional value. In addition, they contain valuable fiber that fruit juice is lacking. Fruit juice can be full of sugar and might even contain preservatives and unnatural ingredients that will have a negative effect on their nutritional value.

84.	You should eat breakfast every day so your body has the energy it needs to function. Studies have shown that people feel better and eat less during the day if they start the morning with a good breakfast. Avoid eating highly processed foods. Make sure your breakfast has some protein in it to help you feel satisfied.

85.   Vitamin K is an advantageous nutrient that you can add to your body on a daily basis. This vitamin is very beneficial in reducing bruises and any imperfections that you may have on the skin. If you suffer from severe acne, vitamin K can help to reduce the redness from your bumps.

86.   The humble cabbage family (including kale, collard and mustard greens), provides us with an especially good buy, nutritionally. If you haven't yet added these to your diet, you should. These dark green leafy vegetables are renowned providers of phosphorus, calcium, iron and carotenoids. Also, they are inexpensive!

87.   Always choose products with the most vitamins listed on the nutrition label. Choosing one product with more vitamins than another similar tasting product, will help your body build up your immune system, strengthen your bones and provide you many more health benefits, over a long period of time.

88.   To replace the junky snacks you might have previously brought into the house, stock up on a variety of easy-to-eat fruits that you can grab when dinner is a ways off and you or your family are hungry. Great examples would be berries, grapes, apples cut into chunks and kept in acidulated water, and small or baby bananas. Keeping the fruit in clear containers in the fridge, or on the counter, will increase its "curb appeal."

89.   Lower your sodium intake by flavoring foods with herbs and spices, rather than salt. By using fresh herbs in everything from sandwiches to vegetables to eggs, you can amp up the flavor without the negative health effects of sodium. Herbs are simple to grow on your kitchen windowsill or porch and therefore, can be easily accessible whenever you need them.

90.   To stay healthy while dieting, choose low calorie but nutrient rich foods. Grapefruit, asparagus, and cantaloupe contain very few calories, but provide your body with many essential vitamins. You should also look for low calorie foods that are high in protein, such as salmon and kidney beans. These will give you the energy you need to get through the day.

91.   People who suffer from diabetes have to deal with nutritional needs that are much more complicated than the regular person. It will help to eat regularly, ensuring that your blood sugar remains within a healthy range. Diabetics should consume copious amounts of fruits and veggies, plus fat free dairy and whole grain staples. They need the discipline to eat around the same time each day.

92.   To reduce the amount of sugar in your diet, try using natural sweeteners instead of white sugar. Honey, molasses, and syrup can sweeten your food without adding as many calories. When you're baking, try substituting fruit juice for some of the sugar. Use fresh fruit to add some sweetness to your cereal in the morning instead of another spoonful of sugar.

93.   If you are searching for a vitamin that helps to reduce depression and sadness, look no further than vitamin B-12. This vitamin is a great addition to your morning arsenal, as it will help to put you in a good mood so that you will have the motivation to exercise and eat well all day.

94.   True yams are very different from sweet potatoes, but are worth seeking out, and are frequently found in ethnic markets. It's got lots of

Vitamin C and B6, in addition to lots of minerals and fiber. They are quite popular baked in their skins or mashed, where their natural sweetness and bright color makes them popular with kids.

95.   When deciding what to eat, keep in mind that you are only eating to gain energy for your body. Eating should not be considered a hobby. When you keep in mind that are only eating to gain energy, you may choose to pass on the unhealthy foods and try to eat foods that will give you the most energy.

96.   When you are thinking about changing your diet you should try to consult with a nutritionist. They are often quite cheap for one or two consultations and they will be able to help you design a meal plan that is perfect for your body type as well as your nutrition goals.

97.   Avoid substituting fruit juices for whole fruits. Whole fruits are fresher and will offer you a higher nutritional value. In addition, they contain valuable fiber that fruit juice is lacking. Fruit juice can be full of sugar and might even contain preservatives and unnatural ingredients that will have a negative effect on their nutritional value.

98.   We all know that eating too much can be a problem, but what about not eating enough? Lots of people think that overeating is the focal point, but they don't understand that not eating enough is dangerous too. Undereating can cause your blood sugar to get too low, which will cause you to crave sweets. Eating small frequent meals throughout the day will help you lose weight and stay healthy.

99.   Plan ahead for healthy nutrition. Keep healthy snacks on hand so that you don't make a poor choice, on the spur of the moment when you get hungry. If the healthy and nutritional choice is the easier one, it becomes a habit to pick that option instead of putting forth the effort to locate an unhealthy item.

100.   Consuming enough Vitamin D is an important part of a healthy, nutritious diet. Vitamin D is a major player in blood clotting. It also helps in bone synthesis. You can find Vitamin D in cabbage, beef liver, and green leafy vegetables. It's also found in smaller amounts in milk, cereals, meats, and eggs.

101.   Many people don't like to bother with breakfast. One reason to focus on good nutrition in the morning is that your brain has literally been fasting all night: You need that boost of energy and protein in the morning to get your brain and body working

quickly for the day. A good protein-and-fruit-based breakfast smoothie will provide a quick way to improve your nutrition profile from the time you wake up in the morning.

102.   It is a great idea to teach your child how to be nutritious if they can get their examples straight from you. If you are eating healthy foods, your child will feel much more inclined to be just like you and eat those same foods. If they see you refusing healthy foods, then they will follow suit.

103.   A great nutritional tip is to set a good example for your child. You want to make healthy choices because - how you eat - will directly influence how your child eats. If you eat unhealthy and your diet is terrible, chances are your child will adopt the same habits.

104.   To naturally detoxify your body, look for foods that are high in soluble fiber. When your body digests soluble fiber, it turns it to water, which makes it ideal for detoxification. Foods rich in this nutrient include carrots, apples, and green peas. These foods also provide your body with essential nutrients, making them a great way to boost your overall health.

105.   To ensure your thyroid gland functions properly, include plenty of iodine in your diet. Iodine is a component of multiple thyroid hormones, including triiodothyronine and thyroxine. Insufficient iodine levels leave your body unable to synthesize thyroid hormones, which means your metabolism cannot be regulated properly. Foods that contain iodine include kelp, eggs, and strawberries.

106.   Don't be sucked in by expensive "super-foods"! Normal food is just fine for nutritional value. Make healthful choices in fresh fruits and veggies, lean meats and fish, legumes, beans and nuts and whole grain breads and cereals at your local market. Use a water purifying pitcher to provide you with plenty of pure water economically. Avoid junk, and eat normal, healthful food in abundance for optimum health.

107.   Always be aware of your sugar intake. Many times people will drink juice thinking it's a nutritional choice, when really it can be filled with sugar. Some juices actually contain more sugar then a can of pop. Read the food labels of everything you eat, and if it has a lot of sugar, skip it.

108.   Breast feed after having a baby. Your body will burn an additional 500 to 800 calories each day to

produce milk. These added calories can get you back to your pre-pregnancy weight much faster. Make sure to eat a healthy balanced diet though, as you will still need a greater calorie intake until you stop breastfeeding.

109.   When pregnant, ensure your diet contains enough vitamin B12. This vitamin helps to cut down on the chances that your little one will have a birth defect. For the most part women really should not worry about being deficient in vitamin B12, however, if you are someone who diets regularly then it should be monitored.

110.   Start your children off right. Early nutrition builds healthy eating habits. Giving in to your childs demands for high sugar, high fat and fried comfort foods will only set them on a path for obesity and malnutrition later on. Insist that they eat fruits, vegetables, healthy low fat proteins and whole grains.

111.   Make a healthy and nutritious dinner with potatoes. Instead of topping with just sour cream, cheese and bacon, try adding lots of fresh and cooked vegetables. Onions, broccoli, tomatoes are all great choices. You can also add black or pinto beans for an added punch of fiber.

112.   Broccoli is a super-food. Broccoli contains tons of minerals, fiber, Vitamins K, A and C and can help to prevent cancer. Steaming or microwaving helps contain nutrients during cooking. When it turns to gray mush, it is not useful.

113.   When trying to diet, an easier way to do it is to add fruit and vegetables rather than trying to remove other foods. Nutritionists recommend 5-9 servings of plants every day, which will get your body the vitamins it needs and satisfy hunger that might otherwise have been filled with fast food.

114.   Good nutrition is the basis for good physical and mental health. You simply can not feel your best if you live on a diet of sugar, fat and salt. Begin thinking of food as fuel and building blocks for your body, as well as material for healthy mental function. If you think like that, you'll see little room for junk food in the picture. Save high-fat, high-sugar and salty splurges for special occasions.

115.   A colorful plate is a healthy plate. Fill at least half of your dinner plate with red, orange, and dark green vegetables, and you are on your way to a well balanced meal packed with vitamins and other nutrients. Add a side dish of fruit to your meal to finish things.

116. Limit the amount of juice and soda that are consumed in your household. While juice does contain some vitamins, it is not a good substitute for eating the whole fruit with the skin. Soda is basically flavored, carbonated water that costs a lot of money. For optimum health you should spend your calories on healthy foods, not on liquid.

117. Mix protein and carbohydrates when you sit down to eat. You'll still get energy from the carbohydrates, but the protein will ensure that there is something in your system besides sugar. Eating a mix of the two this way will keep your blood sugar stable and keep your appetite down.

118. A great tip if you want to live a healthier lifestyle is to eat lean meat. In particular, you want to eat meat that is rich in omega-3 like fish. Lean meat has a lot of protein, which is needed to fuel your muscles and ensure your body operates efficiently.

119. Pay close attention to your meal plan in order to have a better day. If you eat too much, you will not feel good during the day and will put on some extra pounds. This can interfere with normal body processes and can be detrimental to your health.

120. A great way to get a healthy and nutritional start to your day is with a balanced breakfast. Include a

protein source, such as a dairy product, a carbohydrate source such as cereal or toast, and a fruit or vegetable such as a banana. This will keep you from getting hungry later as well.

121.   Calcium is one of the most important things our bodies need to perform optimally. Whether you're nine years old or forty-nine years old, everyone needs calcium. At younger ages, calcium aids in the building of healthy bones. At older ages, our bones begin to deteriorate. Calcium can slow and even stop that process.

122.   Omega 3 fatty acids should be consumed for a healthy heart. These poly unsaturated fatty acids work to lower the triglycerides and increase HDL, the good cholesterol, in your body. Omega 3 fatty acids can also prevent blood from clotting inside your body. Studies also show that consuming Omega 3 fats can help to lower blood pressure.

123.   Consume 600-900 mg of garlic, about 1 fresh clove, daily to help lower your cholesterol. There have been many studies where people have used garlic for health reasons. These studies have proven garlic is extremely beneficial in helping to lower total cholesterol, and in particular, LDL, the bad cholesterol and triglycerides.

124.   Stick to all-natural foods instead of those produced and refined in factories. Many times those foods add items such as extra fats, oils, greases and preservatives that can really harm your body. Try shopping from the parts of the stores where you can purchase produce, healthy protein and other "from the earth" products.

125.   Watch how you prepare your food and see if you can do better. If you are one for frying in oils and fats constantly, you can cook much healthier. Try steaming, baking, broiling and grilling. This will also help to avoid depleting the essential nutrients in your food.

126.   To eat healthier, you should avoid certain kind of meats. Meat is necessary to your diet, but you need to learn how to recognize what kind of meat is good. Stay away from fried chicken or rich sauces and gravy. Healthy meats include red meats such as beef, and poultry.

127.   Senior citizens looking to be as heart-healthy as possible can enjoy a Mediterranean diet. This way of eating includes healthy fats such as those found in olive oil; it also includes plenty of vegetables, seafood, beans, high-fiber grains, and fruits. Studies have shown that the Mediterranean diet, because of

the healthier fats it contains, lowers the risk of heart disease.

128.   To reduce the pain of menstrual cramps, try consuming bromelain. Bromelain is substance found in pineapple. It's a natural muscle relaxer that works similarly to many over the counter drugs. However, because bromelain is a natural substance, its effects can last much longer. Bromelain has also been shown to reduce the number of inflammatory cells in your body.

129.   Crunchy carrots are healthy additions to your diet. Don't forget to add them to your diet. Besides being tasty snacks, they have significant health benefits. There carotene, Vitamin A, minerals, antioxidants and dietary fiber content protect your skin, improve your eyesight and add healthy levels of minerals to your body.

130.   When looking to improve your nutrition with a good source of antioxidants, don't overlook the value of the ever popular pumpkin. The antioxidant in pumpkin comes from beta-carotene. It can give a boost to your immune system function and reduce the risk of cancer and heart disease. Adding pumpkin to your diet also gives you added fiber.

131.   A great nutrition tip is to opt for white meat when you're eating chicken or turkey. Although dark meat may taste good, it is much higher in fat. White meat is leaner and much healthier for you. Stay away from the thighs as well and stick with the breast.

132.   When it is time to eat try to sit down and enjoy your meal. When you eat meals standing up or while on the go your body does not digest all of the food the way that it should be doing and you will have a harder time getting the extra weight off.

133.   When eating at a salad bar, you can make yourself a wonderful nutritious meal. Load up on the dark leafy greens, add some carrots and peppers along with other vegetables that look tasty. Don't pile on thick creamy dressing, or it won't be healthy for you to eat at all.

134.   You don't have to give up your favorite fried foods or sweets to achieve good nutrition in pregnancy, just limit the amount you consume. Substitute some cut up vegetables or a hand full of almonds for just one of your daily sweet treats. Don't feel guilty if you indulge from time to time, but picking a nutritious option instead will benefit your baby in the long run.

135.   Pyroxidine is another of the most important vitamins to the human body. It is involved in such vital functions as production of red blood cells and electrolyte (sodium and potassium, mainly) balance in the blood. It is also important for brain function. Foods that contain it, include grains and seeds.

136.   The drinks one choosing can often be some of the worst things for them nutritionally. Pops, certain juices, and other drinks can be very high in sugars. The sugars in these drinks do not do any good for ones nutrition. Drinking water or healthier minded drinks can be beneficial to ones nutrition.

137.   Rice is part of numerous dishes that people prepare every day. Substituting brown rice for white rice an excellent way to make any rice dish diet-friendly. While white rice is a source of empty carbohydrates, brown rice has fewer calories and is much more filling. Multi-grain rice is also a great option.

138.   Make sure to start each day by eating a nutritious breakfast. This is the most important meal of the day and is much needed fuel to begin the day. Try eating items like oatmeal, low-fat yogurt, smoothies, whole grain toast, whole grain waffles and lean meats. This will not keep you full, but will help keep you full until your next meal.

139.   Even artificial sweeteners can raise your blood sugar and insulin levels in much the same way as sugar. Although they may be lower in calories, they are not necessarily any more healthy. Instead change on how much you depend on sweet things. Start by cutting your sugars in half and work you way to not needing them at all.

140.   One decision regarding nutrition is whether or not to eat meat. A vegetarian diet has long been espoused in the East, less so in the West. There are voices which show the nutritional deficiencies of a diet without meat. There are vegetarian advocates who show ways to make up these deficiencies-- without eating meat. Consider both and decide for yourself!

141.   Making sure that you're giving your body the proper nutrition that it needs can be hard at times. Taking a daily multivitamin can help ensure that some of your nutritional needs are always met. Many daily multivitamins provide a full day's worth of several vitamins and minerals that your body needs in one small pill.

142.   When considering your nutrition intake at a fast food restaurant, what may seem like the lesser of two evils may not always be the healthiest. Chicken

often times ends up having more sodium and calories than a burger due to toppings such as ranch and additions such as bacon. If you feel as though you must satisfy a fast food craving, be sure to check the nutrition chart first.

143.   When considering your nutrition, be sure to watch out for foods that may appear healthy but end up being quite the opposite. There can be a lot of hidden fat and sodium in otherwise healthy looking snacks. Smoothies can end up having a lot of fat calories and sugar depending on the ingredients used. Energy bars can be a hidden source of a large amount of calories. Fat free foods can contain the same amount of calories as regular versions.

144.   Try not to use dessert as a reward for eating healthy. If a child sees dessert as a reward, they're going to think that it is the best food. This will only reinforce their desire to have sweets. If you want to use dessert as a reward, try offering fruits and other healthy foods.

145.   Fortify your food choices with a naturally found nutrient called inulin. Inulin can be found in garlic, artichokes and leeks. It is a powerful carbohydrate and not only will it help you shed pounds, it can help prevent digestive problems. Garlic is an

excellent immune booster as well. Try blanching garlic to reduce odor if you are worried about garlic breath or opt to take a odorless garlic supplement.

146.   When working in a busy office, it is common for one or more of your colleges to have a tempting bowl of candy for anyone to eat. Bring your own snacks to work so you can stay strong. Fill individual snack bags with single servings of rice cakes or some almonds to keep you going.

147.   To lower the amount of tissue damage done by free radicals, include copper in your diet. Superoxide dismutase, an enzyme essential in removing free radicals from the body, is dependent on copper to function properly. A copper deficiency severely limits your body's ability to fight free radicals. Foods high in copper include cashews, sweet potatoes, and oysters.

148.   If you are eating at a restaurant, and you are offered fries, skip them. They are loaded with fat and salt, which will make you feel bloated, and greasy. Instead, order a side salad or some fresh fruit. When you make healthier choices like these, you will end up feeling better knowing you are taking care of yourself.

149.   Prepackaged foods should be the exception not the rule. Make your food from raw ingredients. Even boxed dinners that require you to add your own meat or other ingredients still contain heavily processed ingredients and spices. Look up some tasty recipes on line and commit to making four of them a week for dinners.

150.   Drinking at least 4 glasses of water a day helps your daily nutrition despite the fact that water carries absolutely no caloric content or vitamins. Water simply helps the digestion and interacts with your body in many different ways. Water is both utilized by your body for chemical reactions and to flush the system of elements that are toxic at certain concentrations.

151.   When trying to diet, an easier way to do it is to add fruit and vegetables rather than trying to remove other foods. Nutritionists recommend 5-9 servings of plants every day, which will get your body the vitamins it needs and satisfy hunger that might otherwise have been filled with fast food.

152.   Milk is the best form of liquid protein you can give you body. Packed full of protein, vitamin D and other important nutrients, milk is a natural, affordable drink, that everyone should take advantage of. Instead of using protein shakes to

bulk up, consider drinking two or three glasses of milk every day, instead.

153.   An unknown boon to many, studies have shown that red wine is actually a healthy choice. Compared to white wine, red wine has less sugar and more healthy nutrients. Nutritionists believe that drinking one glass of red wine per day may increase your life expectancy. The same idea applies to dark chocolate.

154.   For young kids you want to make eating healthy fun for them. If they don't like vegetables, try cooking them differently or serving them with a sauce your child likes. You can also try cutting foods into different shapes like stars, dinosaurs, etc. so that the kid can have fun while eating healthy.

155.   An effective method in getting your child to try something new is not by talking about how it tastes, but by discussing what it looks like and feels like. This can help you child to become intererested in the food, possibly enough to give it a taste.

156.   Be aware of what you drink. Avoid any drinks that contain alcohol or sugar, replacing them with water, low-fat milk or tea. Sugary drinks are packed full of empty calories that add no nutritional value to your diet. Drinking one sugary drink a day can

cause you to put on unnecessary weight, and increases your risk of developing high blood pressure.

157.   If you want your vegetable dishes to contain less fat, cook them with water, not oil. Steaming and boiling vegetables are tasty and better for you than fried ones. If oil just has to be used, think about using small amounts of vegetable oil rather than butter.

158.   Part of getting good nutrition is eating your fruits and vegetables. You should be eating around 5 servings every day. Fruits and vegetables are loaded with fiber, vitamins and beneficial antioxidants. Eating like this will fill you up fast, and they are low in calories, so if you are watching your weight, they are also the perfect food.

159.   Use pureed fruit for a healthy substitute for commercial meat sauces. Fruit that is in season is more than affordable. You can puree up everything from apples to pineapples to marinate your fish, poultry, pork or beef. It works when you are barbecuing and even inside on the range or oven.

160.   Not everyone likes to talk about it, but everybody knows it: Fiber keeps your regular. Meeting your recommended daily allowance of fiber

is easier than ever with commercially prepared over-the-counter fiber supplements, not to mention the abundance of fiber found naturally in popular foods like oats, whole grains, lettuce, fresh spinach, and most other vegetables. Getting enough fiber also helps to lower your risk of developing heart disease and certain types of diabetes.

161.   When you are looking for something to snack on, open the refrigerator. You will most likely find choices that are more healthy than anything you can find in your pantry or freezer. Try filling your fridge with fruits and vegetables so you always have easy access to a snack.

162.   Avoid foods that contain monosodium glutamate. Commonly known as "MSG", this is a food additive used by many restaurants and food manufacturers to enhance the flavor of food. It adds no nutritional value. Many people experience adverse symptoms like headaches, nausea, and heart palpitations after consuming foods with MSG. To avoid possible reaction, you should avoid foods containing MSG altogether.

163.   Limit the consumption of meats. There is never the need to eat a steak that is larger than eight ounces. It is too hard for your body to digest and will end up being more toxic than nutritional. Stick

with meats that are white and choose a meal that includes three to six ounces of the white meats.

164.   While vacationing, don't forget the importance of eating healthy. Vacation is the best, and worst, time to indulge. It's easy to get off your healthy eating kick and fill yourself with junk food. Try to incorporate some fresh and local fruits and vegetables into your meals. Don't over do the alcohol or sweets. A treat once in awhile is great, but remember moderation. Your body will thank you for it.

165.   When trying to diet, an easier way to do it is to add fruit and vegetables rather than trying to remove other foods. Nutritionists recommend 5-9 servings of plants every day, which will get your body the vitamins it needs and satisfy hunger that might otherwise have been filled with fast food.

166.   Great, nutritious fruit snack choices that you and your whole family will enjoy include, sliced apples with peanut butter, grapes that have been rinsed, allowed to dry and then frozen, fresh fruit and yogurt. Always try to use fresh fruit instead of canned, but remember that even canned fruit is more nutritious than processed snack cakes and other poor snacking choices.

167.   Control yourself when dining outside. Splurging in a social environment may be very tempting, especially when out with friends who don't follow a particular diet plan. This can be counterproductive because it both indulges your negative eating habits but also sets up a precedent for breaking your dietary rules as well.

168.   To avoid eating too much food at mealtime when dieting, use smaller plates, bowls and cups. It is instinct to fill up your plate so if you use smaller dishes, you will eat less food. Your mind will also let your stomach know you are full since you see a full plate when eating.

169.   Whether or not you are vegetarian or a meat eater, protein is a very important part of your diet. You should eat protein at every single meal to keep your blood insulin or blood sugar levels balanced. Eating too many carbohydrates and not enough protein, can give you an energy high, now and an energy crash, later.

170.   When considering nutrition for your child, be sure to not deprive them of sweets or other dessert type foods. It is important that this be included as part of the meal, so that dessert is seen as a normal food, not something that should be desired more

than the meal itself. Be sure to work in as many healthy desserts as possible.

171.   Eating organic foods can be an effective way of increasing the nutritional content of your diet. Mounting scientific evidence shows that organic foods are higher in nutrients, and lower in nitrates. Organic building blocks form healthier foods, just as Mother Nature intended. Take one taste and you will understand.

172.   Shopping more frequently for produce can reduce waste and increase the likelihood of actually eating fresh fruits and vegetables. Lots of people purchase their groceries once a week and sometimes forget to eat their fresh produce. If you stop by the store slightly more often, things won't spoil as often and you'll get into the habit of eating more fresh produce in no time.

173.   Beans, beans what a wonderful food. Studies have shown that eating beans can reduce your chances of developing heart disease and could also prevent breast cancer. These great properties are thanks to beans' high protein, vitamin, and fiber content. To reduce the chance of indigestion, add them to your diet gradually.

174.   Eating the right diet that supports exercise levels and gives the body the required materials to rebuild itself, is a key component to physical fitness. Having the right amount of protein will allow for muscle growth. Providing enough carbohydrates will give the body fuel for the day. The right diet makes a big difference.

175.   A great nutritional tip is to start eating prawns. Prawns are loaded with quality nutrition, including protein, essential fats, and alanine. Alanine is an amino acid, and it's important because it produces carnosine, which is an antioxidant that helps the body respond better to the acid produced by exercise.

176.   To increase the effectiveness of vitamin supplements, include plenty of manganese in your diet. Manganese has been shown to help your body absorb a variety of vitamins and minerals. Foods rich in manganese include pineapple, soybeans, and brown rice. Consuming these foods about an hour before you take any vitamins w,ill help your body take full advantage of them.

177.   The olive oil in your pantry can be a valuable addition to your skin care routine by fighting dryness. Olive oil is gentle and effective in sealing in moisture on your face and hands. It also provides a

helping of antioxidants to combat aging. A thin layer twice a day is all you need.

178.   Slow down when you're eating. It takes up to half an hour from the time you start eating until the time you start feeling full. So if you are eating slowly, in half an hour you'll feel full and you won't have stuffed yourself and overeaten to do it.

179.   If you have to have coffee in the mornings, the best thing you can do is to have it black, but if you must have it sweet and creamy, you do have an option. You can put skim milk and sugar substitute in it and it will be just as satisfying.

180.   When you are really craving something salty, many types of nuts have very high nutritional value, but you have to keep in mind that they also have very high calories. If you take a few pistachios or walnuts and put them on a plate with some low calorie cheese you will have a great satisfying snack.

181.   Avoid all processed foods at all costs. These foods are simply bad for you in every way. Eat foods that are as close to natural as you can get. Whole grains, whole, raw or lightly cooked vegetables and fruits, and organic, humanely raised meats are your best bets for the best in nutrition.

182.   Keep a ceramic or glass kettle of pure water with a bit of honey and a fresh squeezed lemon or lime warming on the back of your stove during the winter months. You can drink cup after cup of this healthful beverage to keep cold and chill at bay and provide you with all the pure water you need to stay healthy and strong.

183.   Explore bean and legume dips and spreads, as nutritious alternatives to high calorie, low nutrition dips and spreads. Refried beans, hummus (made from garbanzo beans) and lentil soup make great, healthful alternates to common snack dips. Salsa and pico de gallo are also excellent, healthy choices. Remember to dip with fresh veggies instead of chips, at least half the time.

184.   Try to incorporate more raw foods into your diet, as they are better for you. Processing or cooking food reduces the amount of vitamins and nutrients it contains. This is especially the case for fruits and veggies.

185.   If you suffer from hot flashes related to menopause, studies have shown that eating soy foods can help. Consuming soy will help prevent hot flashes in women going through menopause. In Japan where soy foods are much more common,

the women rarely suffer from menopause symptoms like the women in the United States.

186.   Try adding more foods to your diet for more variety and more nutrients. There are endless healthy options you can make when you have access to many different types of foods. variety keeps you from getting bored with your diet and also prevents you from turning to unhealthy food options.

187.   Be aware of what chemicals are in your food. This is generally why it's best to stick to natural food like natural produce and fresh proteins and natural grain options. You should avoid these like you would anything else hazardous because they can slow down your metabolic rate and harm your diet.

188.   Many people don't like to bother with breakfast. One reason to focus on good nutrition in the morning is that your brain has literally been fasting all night: You need that boost of energy and protein in the morning to get your brain and body working quickly for the day. A good protein-and-fruit-based breakfast smoothie will provide a quick way to improve your nutrition profile from the time you wake up in the morning.

189.   A great tip to live a healthier lifestyle is to calculate how many calories you need on a daily

basis. The amount of calories you need every day varies with every person depending on many different factors such as sex, weight, height, body type, etc. Once you calculate your daily caloric needs, you can count your calories to ensure you stay at your daily need.

190.   Make sure that you get enough Vitamin-A in your diet. The fat-soluble vitamin aids skin repair. Deficiencies can cause dry, cracked, flaky, infected skin. Foods high in Vitamin-A include spinach, carrots, liver and apricots. Try to avoid artificial Vitamin-A supplements. Taking excessive amounts of the vitamin can have harmful effects.

191.   It is important to include food which provide selenium in your diet. Selenium is a mineral with antioxidant properties that contribute to the elasticity of tissue and help to prevent the aging of skin prematurely. Also, selenium is helpful in protecting your skin from the sun. Foods that contain a significant amount selenium include tuna, eggs, garlic, wheat germ and brown rice.

192.   A good nutritional tip is to make sure you get enough potassium in your diet. Bloating may occur when you're consuming too much sodium, and not enough potassium. Some foods that contain potassium include bananas, fish, and cantaloupe.

The more salt you consume, the more potassium you'll need.

193.   Make a salad for dinner. You can add chicken, fish, or other lean meats, as well as lots of fresh veggies like carrots, corn, peas, tomatoes and even throw in some strawberries, mandarin oranges or pineapple for some sweet pizazz. Making a salad the entree will keep you from using a high calorie and carbohydrate like pasta instead.

194.   Smell the aroma of apples, peppermint, or bananas. Certain foods such as the ones mentioned are known to suppress appetite. Some people believe that these smells actually deceive the body into thinking that the person is eating or has eaten food. Suppressing your appetite will help you keep a healthy weight.

195.   A healthy diet will help to boost your immune system. By boosting your body's immune system your body will be able to fight against the impurities that cause skin problems. Just keeping track of what you are putting in your body and making sure that what you put in your body boosts the immune system.

196.   High fructose corn syrup, sugar, and other forms of carbohydrates are all essentially the same

when it comes to nutrition. They might react in a different manner with the body, diffusing sugar faster, but they all carry similar calorie contents and behave like sugars. Starches like bread and pasta provide a large portion of carbohydrates which allows you to store up energy in fat cells.

197.   Vegetables like celery and lettuce have high fiber content. Fiber content is good for your bowel system because it provides roughage, indigestible material that passes through the body and helps things pass through. They also have very low calorie content due to the nature of their stem and leaf like qualities. The plants have very low sugar content, and are great for losing weight.

198.   Find snack foods that provide protein first, then carbs or sugar. Veggies and fruits make healthy snacks, but maintaining blood sugar throughout the day requires protein as well. Add nuts or cheese to your snakcs to get the maximum amount of value out of your snacking with more energy and improved mental focus.

199.   When considering sides for your meal in a restaurant you should consider the steamed, grilled, boiled, or raw options that are available. Steamed vegetables are much healthier than fried versions. Many restaurants will give you the option to get a

salad if they do not have any options for vegetables that are not fried or swimming in butter.

200.   You should never skip meals when you are in the process of trying to lose some excess weight. While it may seem you would lose weight from this, most people usually end up overeating during the following meal because they are hungry from the lack of food at the earlier time.

201.   Try to substitute healthy alternatives for fatty or sugary foods you enjoy. For example, instead of a bowl of ice cream, you can have some yogurt with fruit. Instead of french fries, try half of a baked potato. You don't have to cut out all the good tasting food in your life, just make healthier choices about what the tasty things you do eat.

202.   People over 50 need to maintain good nutrition by ensuring they get enough vitamin D and calcium. This is because, as people age, their bones become more brittle. Calcium will help reduce bone loss, and vitamin D helps the bones absorb the calcium. People aged 50 and over should boost their calcium intake either via non-fat dairy products or through supplements.

203.   Try not to use dessert as a reward for eating healthy. If a child sees dessert as a reward, they're

going to think that it is the best food. This will only reinforce their desire to have sweets. If you want to use dessert as a reward, try offering fruits and other healthy foods.

204.　Keep a healthy snack in your vehicle, your desk, and your purse. You can reach for it instead of taking that piece of cake the secretary brought into the office. You'll know the calorie content up front and not be so disgusted with yourself that you give up on staying on your health plan that day.

205.　Nutrition is one of the key components to proper weight control. Knowing what to eat and what to avoid can help you lose weight or maintain your current weight if you have reached your goal. Fresh fruits and vegetables are great snacks that can help keep weight off and give you what you need in nutrition when it comes to vitamins and minerals.

206.　Pack your lunch. Rather than going to a fast food restaurant for lunch, bring your own. Use a variety of bread for healthy sandwiches, such as wholemeal rolls, ciabatta or pita bread. Choose fillings that are high in protein such as chicken or tuna. A healthy alternative to a sandwich is a flask of soup, and always include a piece of fresh fruit or some sliced raw vegetables.

207.   Vitamins play a very important role in our life. Some of them can be synthesized by our body, but most of them should be included in our daily food. It is a good practice to eat lots of fresh fruits, vegetables, soy, whole grain bakery products, nuts and beans. Without these building blocks we become sick.

208.   If you are looking for a tasty addition to your meal that will provide filling, choose beans. Beans are essential to help the flow of foods through your body, and have a lot of nutrients that are vital. Also, beans contain protein, which help to convert fat to muscle, reducing your weight.

209.   Make sure to add foods rich in choline to your nutritional, pregnancy diet, in order to boost fetal brain development. When you are pregnant, your reserve of choline is used up quickly, so it is especially important to include eggs in your daily nutrition routine. It is important to prepare the whole egg because the choline is found in the yolk.

210.   A good way to get your whole family to eat their veggies is to make a pizza loaded with them. Include their favorite toppings like cheese and pepperoni, but then pile on the tomatoes, olives, onions, and other pizza friendly vegetable toppings. Don't let them pick it off either.

211.   To maintain optimum nutrition in your diet it is important to get a wide variety of colors on your plate. The different colors really are different nutrients your body needs. Try to get at least three different colors into every meal. Try greens like kale, grapes, and cucumbers; reds like tomatoes, strawberries, and chilis; oranges like sweet potatoes, fall squashes, and carrots; light colors like cauliflower, potatoes, turnips, and whole grains; as well as other bright colors you see in blueberries, mangoes, avocados, peppers, and pineapple. Eating a diversity of colors will keep your nutrition balanced.

212.   By buying produce at a local farmers market or from a farm stand that one knows of in the area, an individual can get a variety of locally grown fruits and vegetables. Not only will one be getting the nutritional benefits from the fruits and vegetables but they will be supporting their local farmers.

213.   Reduce the refined foods in your diet. Refined foods are high in sugars, empty carbohydrates, and fats. They contain less nutritional value per calorie than unrefined foods. Avoiding them can lead to a healthier diet and lifestyle. Your best bet is to stick with raw, fresh foods whenever possible.

214.   Although fitness and nutrition are not the same thing they are in the same area - health. If you want to improve your overall health level you should consider exercise as well. This will actually help you to stay motivated about your eating habits as your body will start to crave healthier foods.

215.   When your goal is proper nutrition, you need to learn to how to eat a properly balanced diet. When planning your daily meals, you need to incorporate the right nutritional components. Aim for 50% carbs, 20% protein and 30% fat for every meal you eat.

216.   Good nutrition will give your body what it needs, but only exercise can shape and strengthen your body. These factors deal more with mental strength, rather than physical. What this means is that your attitude and drive has as much to do with your success when exercising as your physical strength. Understanding this will help you to maximize your body physically and mentally.

217.   Eat more fish for your health and for your brain. Fish are high in DHA which has been shown to improve your memory, vocabulary and prowess in nonverbal tasks. DHA may also reduce the risk of Alzheimer's. Fish is also a great source of protein

and the Omega-3 fatty acids may be beneficial to your heart health.

218.   Vitamin A is an important part of a healthy diet. You can get it from such foods as dairy products, eggs, beef liver, dark greens, and orange fruit and vegetables. Vitamin A is necessary for for vision, particularly night vision. It also aids in the repair of bone and tissue.

219.   Add some avocados into your daily nutritional diet. They are rich in many nutrients. Avocados contain monounsaturated fats that help reduce the level of cholesterol. They are also high in potassium, an important mineral in stabilizing blood pressure. Avocados are a good source of folate, which is important for a healthy heart.

220.   Organic food is much in the news these days and many of us are paying attention, as we should. Eating organically grown foods maximizes the nutrients we receive. One reason is that the soil on an organic farm is richer in the nutrients we need, which then imparts these nutrients into the food that we eat.

221.   You want to try and keep a routine with your kid's meal times. Try to serve meals and snacks at roughly the same time every day. Let your child

have juice or milk at meal times only, and drink water the rest of the time. If they drink juice and milk all day, they may not have an appetite later.

222.   Dairy products are a great source of calcium and vitamin D, which help to build bone mass. Additionally, studies have shown that 1,000 milligrams of calcium per day, can help you lose weight, particularly around your midsection. Low-fat yogurt is highly versatile and can be used as a substitute for sour cream, mayonnaise and even cheese.

223.   If you are on a vegetarian or vegan diet, you need to find plenty of ways to incorporate protein into your diet. Protein is an important building block for muscle development, and it is very easy for vegetarians to lose muscle mass when they reduce the meat and animal products from their diet.

224.   Sometimes people fail when trying to lose weight because they allow themselves to get so busy, and don't have the time or energy to cook anything. Make an emergency kit for times like these that is filled with healthy foods like nuts, fruits and veggies. Take that with you wherever you go, and if you are hungry you will have something to

eat that does not include a drive through and extra pounds.

225.   Avoid drinking your calories in liquid form. Drinks with a great deal of calories, such as milk, energy drinks and fruit juice can give you a large amount of calories without satiating your hunger. Sodas, beer, drink mixes and shakes are full of empty calories and provide no nutritional content whatsoever.

226.   If you're working on addressing your nutrition concerns, make sure you don't villainize any food groups! Most things are okay in moderation, which means that, cutting carbohydrates out of your diet, is wholly unnecessary. Enjoy your pasta and bread in moderation and you'll enjoy long-term energy, if you're maintaining your protein intake, as well.

227.   Sometimes, it is hard to stay on track with a healhty diet while traveling. There are times that you may have to stop at a fast food restaurant. If you do, there are a few things you can do to cut calories. First, order your burger with no cheese or condiments. Also, if possible, choose grilled meats or a salad bar.

228.   Always try to eat local, seasonal produce. Produce that is in season and local, is fresh and has

had less opportunity to lose valuable nutrients. It is, therefore, the healthiest option, full of valuable vitamins and minerals. Shopping your local farmers market can be a great way to find out what is in season and available locally.

229.   When it comes to nutrition, you want to make sure you are constantly keeping an eye on the latest information available to you. With science always learning new things about what is healthy and unhealthy for you, you want to try your best to always, be informed. You never know, something that you think could be helping you today could actually end up harming you in the future, so try your best to stay informed.

230.   Any time that you eat anything, you should remove it from its original packaging. It is much easier to eat an entire bag of chips when they are left in the bag. If you put half of a bag on a plate, you will probably be satisfied after just half a bag.

231.   Try to eliminate the gluten out of your diet. It has been noticed that those with an allergy to gluten seem to end up feeling much better. It leaves them with a clearer head, more energetic, not as bloated, and all around healthier. Try substituting millet, quinoa or amaranth when you have those carb cravings.

232.   Feed your body throughout the day with foods that maximize your energy and health. Three meals and two snacks or even five small "meals" which consist of fresh, organic foods will keep your system functioning at peak levels. Consistent fueling allows for a higher, more consistent metabolism which in turn keeps your weight down.

233.   Eat nuts for a snack instead of crackers. Even though nuts are higher in fat content, eating only a small amount can satisfy your hunger for a longer period of time. Crackers are mainly carbohydrates. You will need to eat more of that to satisfy your hunger over the same period of time, leading to eating more calories. So, in the long run, nuts are better snacks.

234.   It may sound like a broken record but when it comes to nutrition, pull out that food pyramid you were given in elementary school. This will ensure that you get the proper combination of starches, proteins, carbs, and other essential elements of a healthy diet. If you are looking to be a productive member of society, or just of the workplace, being well nourished is the first step.

235.   Try to substitute healthy alternatives for fatty or sugary foods you enjoy. For example, instead of a

bowl of ice cream, you can have some yogurt with fruit. Instead of french fries, try half of a baked potato. You don't have to cut out all the good tasting food in your life, just make healthier choices about what the tasty things you do eat.

236.   Make sure that you are getting enough vitamin E in your diet. Vitamin E is a great antioxidant that helps maintain the health of cell membranes. It has potential benefits in the protection of the heart against disease. Vitamin E is also important to the health of your eyes and plays a role in the prevention of cataracts.

237.   When considering a diet that provides an adequate nutrition level, be sure to schedule regular checkups with your doctor. This will ensure not only that you are doing well with your current nutrition intake, but will also aid in making good choices for your future. Most insurance plans should make it affordable to keep a close eye on your health.

238.   To receive the benefits of antioxidants, you don't have to drink exotic fruit juices. Tomatoes, one of the most common foods, contain loads of these beneficial antioxidants and they also have plenty of vitamins, like C and A. Tomatoes can be enjoyed in various ways. Cherry tomatoes are great

for snacking, while large tomatoes can be used in sandwiches, soups, sauces and many other uses.

239.   One fundamental starting point for good nutrition is to take a daily multivitamin. Although you should not rely on multivitamins for all your nutritional needs, it's helpful to think of a multivitamin as insurance against the nutrients you may not have taken in that day. Also, be aware that multivitamins are available for a wide variety of ages and needs (kids, teens, seniors, prenatal, etc.) and choose one that's right for you.

240.   To cure insomnia through your diet, eat foods that contain magnesium or melatonin. Magnesium works as a natural muscle relaxant, while melatonin helps your body to regulate sleep. Bananas, cherries, and hazelnuts are just a few examples of foods rich in these nutrients. Try making them a part of your last meal or snack of the day.

241.   Read and understand the labels on the food you buy. The nutrition labels list the serving size, the calories, the fat, the sodium, the cholesterol, the carbohydrate, the protein and the vitamin content of each serving. Using this information you can calculate how much you have to eat from each type of food.

242.   The olive oil in your pantry can be a valuable addition to your skin care routine by fighting dryness. Olive oil is gentle and effective in sealing in moisture on your face and hands. It also provides a helping of antioxidants to combat aging. A thin layer twice a day is all you need.

243.   Nutrition experts have recommended that if you increase your carbohydrate intake it can have a positive effect on your overall diet. Since carbohydrates give your body loads of energy per serving, it is certainly a great way to compliment your current diet. It also tends to burn off much easier than fatty foods do.

244.   Avoid drinking your calories in liquid form. Drinks with a great deal of calories, such as milk, energy drinks and fruit juice can give you a large amount of calories without satiating your hunger. Sodas, beer, drink mixes and shakes are full of empty calories and provide no nutritional content whatsoever.

245.   When you go shopping, have a list of planned meals. Going to a store with a specific list will help you not to deviate from the foods you should be eating. This will also make sure that you have all the ingredients on hand to make the right kinds of

foods when you're at home instead of ordering take out.

246.   Do not exclude any food group from your diet. Many weight loss diets support the removal of entire food groups, such as fats or carbohydrates, from the diet. This is a bad mistake as the body needs all the nutrients-vitamins, trace elements, minerals and fiber- that it gets from all food groups.

247.   Eat smaller, more nutritious meals throughout the day. Eating smaller-portioned meals that are several hours apart five or six times a day not only helps with digestion, but also helps to keep your weight down. Keeping your weight down can prevent diseases like diabetes and hypertension. Eating more frequently also helps you to feel less hungry, making it unlikely that you will binge on unhealthy foods.

248.   When it comes to nutrition, we all seem to have trouble doing it properly. Our problem areas vary though and sometimes, we need help identifying these problems. Look at your eating habits and decide which one you pick. Is it the salad or the cheeseburger? The soda or bottled water? The healthy choices are obvious and if you don't pick them as often as you should, that may be your problem.

249.   If you are concerned about healthy nutrition, you will want to look into the growing movement for locally grown food. By buying produce from local small farms you get a fresher product. It hasn't been shipped across country in refrigerated cars! If organically grown, it won't be laden with pesticides.

250.   Allow your children to help you prepare meals. The more involved children are in the process, the more likely they are to eat the meal. This is especially true for things they may not want to try, such as vegetables. It may not make them like broccoli, but it might make them more likely to taste it.

251.   One of the hardest, but most rewarding, things to do in transitioning to a healthy diet is conquering an addiction to unhealthy junk food. Having eaten junk food for a long time, many people have become overly accustomed to its convenience and taste. After switching to a healthy diet, you may still experience pangs and cravings for junk food. You need to redirect these cravings toward healthier alternatives.

252.   When you are craving a glass of fruit juice, you should consider having a small piece of fresh fruit instead. This will curb your craving and it will also

keep you full for much longer. If you must drink fruit juice, try to drink a diet or 100 percent natural version.

253.   When you are trying to decide what to have for dinner, remember that you should have equal amounts of vegetable and grains on your plate. You will be able to get full without eating too much of the calorie-ridden grains. This is because a cup of grains has about 200 calories and the veggies have just 50 or so.

254.   Request a special meal on an airplane to be served first. Airlines usually offer special meals, such as vegetarian or kosher. The people who ask for these are generally served before anyone else. Be careful though, sometimes the meal may take longer to prepare, and you will end up being the last to eat.

255.   If you are tired of boring dishes on your diet that do not contain flavor, add chili pepper sauce to your meal. This will give you the vibrant kick that you need and is also one of the healthiest additives that you can use in your meals when you are dieting.

256.   Make sure you're not forcing your child to eat everything that's on their plate. If you force them to keep eating after they're full, you'll encourage them to overeat. This can lead to problems like obesity

and diabetes down the road. Respect your child's wishes when they say they've had enough.

257.   Always try to have sugarless chewing gum on hand since chewing that can help satisfy sweet cravings and general food cravings. When you get hungry, popping a piece of gum in your mouth actually seems to take the food cravings from you right away and you can wait to eat until it is time for your next meal.

258.   A golden rule is to try not to eat anything that has more than four grams of sugar per serving. This will save a lot of calories and it is particularly helpful for you to follow this rule if you are unfortunate enough to be stricken with diabetes.

259.   A commonly overconsumed mineral in the modern American diet is sodium. While a certain amount of sodium in the diet is vital to continued nervous system function, it is important to not eat too much, as it can lead to high blood pressure. The easiest place to cut it out is with eliminating fast food.

260.   Don't eat poorly during the weekends. Some people believe it is ok to drop their diet or healthy meal plan on the weekends. By eating junk foods over the weekend, you are increasing your chances

of high cholesterol and heart disease as well as undoing any work you have put into your diet.

261. Be sure to drink plenty of pure water. You should drink eight 8 ounce glasses a day. Surprisingly, you may find it easier to drink warm water than cold water. Try a mug of pure water heated to the temperature of a warm beverage or tea. You may find this to be a very enjoyable and relaxing beverage.

262. Eat smaller meals every three to four hours. Many people dislike having to stop what they are doing to eat something, so they end up sskipping breakfast, eating lunch late and then overeating at dinner time becuae they are famished. Find mor efficient ways to prepare quick, healthy meals so that you can get the food in your system. This keeps your blood sugar stable, gives you more energy and maintains your mental focus.

263. Realize that some fruits or vegetables only provide starch-like nutrition. Bananas, for example, are very high in starch but do not necessarily provide the vitamins that humans require in their nutrition. Eating a single banana will not provide the correct amount of vitamins and thus a variety of other fruits are needed to get your total nutritional value.

264. When shopping for food, try to stick to the perimeter; or around the edges of the store. This is usually where the fresh produce is, as well as the meats and dairy products. These are the things to stick to in a healthy diet. By sticking to the perimeter, you'll only buy things that support a healthy diet.

265. While nutritional supplements like protein shakes, vitamin tablets, and other products can be beneficial to your health, it's important to remember that relying on them can be unhealthy and expensive. If you take a lot of these supplements, try to find one food that can act as a natural alternative.

266. It is a great idea to teach your child how to be nutritious if they can get their examples straight from you. If you are eating healthy foods, your child will feel much more inclined to be just like you and eat those same foods. If they see you refusing healthy foods, then they will follow suit.

267. Nuts contain good, natural oils that nourish your skin, nails, hair and body. Be sure to choose natural, unsalted nuts (walnuts, pecans, almonds, cashews, Brazil nuts, peanuts, etc.) to snack on instead of candies, chips and other empty foods.

Nuts are a healthful, nourishing, skin-friendly alternative to mass produced snacks, that damage your health and your skin.

268. Improve the overall quality of your diet by only eating organic products or raw vegetables. These foods are great because they will supply just the nutrients that your skin needs, and nothing extra that will yield fat or irritation. Additionally, you will feel better during the day and energetic while working or at school.

269. To cleanse your colon, look for nutrient rich foods that are rich in fiber. Fiber works as a natural laxative, making it a perfect choice for colon cleansing. To keep your health optimal, you should be sure to consume plenty of nutrients while you cleanse. Foods like green peas, spinach, and kidney beans will cleanse your colon while providing your body with vitamins and minerals.

270. A great nutrition tip is to customize your diet to your body type. Not everyone has the same body type. Some people are more sensitive to carbohydrates and will gain weight just by looking at them, while others can eat anything they want and will never gain any weight.

271.   To naturally reduce your levels of stress, eat foods that contain folic acid. Folic acid works as a mood stabilizer, and can leave you feeling calmer and more relaxed. Examples of foods rich in folic acid include avocado, lentils, and dark leafy greens. Consuming folic acid also reduces your risk for depression.

272.   Don't be sucked in by expensive "super-foods"! Normal food is just fine for nutritional value. Make healthful choices in fresh fruits and veggies, lean meats and fish, legumes, beans and nuts and whole grain breads and cereals at your local market. Use a water purifying pitcher to provide you with plenty of pure water economically. Avoid junk, and eat normal, healthful food in abundance for optimum health.

273.   If you want to add a little variety to your fruits, try dipping them in unsweetened applesauce. Applesauce is great for dipping most of your fruits in. It can add a little bit of variety to your snacks, which will help you from getting bored with eating the same things, all of the time.

274.   If you are having a hard time making sense of the body's complex nutritional needs, you probably are not alone. Consider scheduling an appointment with a licensed nutritionist. These professionals

have years and years experience working with all types of people with all types of specific nutritional needs. A proscribed nutritional plan can make a world of difference in the way you look and feel, but only if you follow it.

275.   Going out to eat, but mindful of nutrition? If you're in the mood to order something high in calories and fat, ask your waiter to divide your meal in half in the kitchen. Your waiter can put half of your meal in a "to go" container, and only bring the other half on your plate. This will help you keep yourself on track with your consumption of calories and fat. It will also let you enjoy some of the good things you love. And you'll get to enjoy it again, for leftover!

276.   Buy lots of frozen vegetables for your freezer so that you always have some on hand. These are great to incorporate into any meal, easy to stir fry and serve as a side or as a main dish with chicken or beef. If you use frozen vegetables instead of fresh ones (for this particular tactic), you needn't worry about wasting money on food that spoils before you get a chance to eat it.

277.   Many people these days like to eat lots of cold water predatory fish, such as swordfish, salmon, and tuna, because they are relatively firm-fleshed and

several are mild-tasting. They also have the advantage of being nutritious and easy to prepare, because they are not as bony. However, they do contain mercury.

278.   A mineral that is extremely rich to add to your diet plan is zinc. Zinc is one of the most powerful antioxidants on the market, as it will help to break down the toxins and free radicals in your body. This will reduce fat and make you feel better as the day wears on.

279.   Cook your own meals. By preparing your own meals at home instead of eating out, you can more easily control the calories contained in your meal. You are able to make healthy ingredient swaps and keep tabs on how much fat and salt are added to the dishes.

280.   If you want to eat more nutritious foods at home and away, you live in very propitious times. Although our markets are filled with an endless array of nutrient-poor foods, you can also choose from a wide variety of much healthier options than were previously available, from low-carb high-fiber tortillas to power-packed super fruit smoothies. For people too busy to cut up vegetables for work lunches, you can purchase little packages of precut fresh veggies and dip. In many ways, while it has

become harder to dodge all the unhealthy choices, it has also become exponentially more convenient to find better nutritional choices.

281.   Look at the ingredients in the food you eat. If you can't pronounce the ingredients, don't buy it. Sticking to foods whose ingredients you can pronounce means that you will be eating in a much healthier way. Those other foods are loaded with preservatives and other things that do not help your body.

282.   Make meals enjoyable and fun to help persuade your picky or nervous eater to try a healthier diet. If your child is wary of certain foods, try cutting them into fun shapes or serve them with a favorite sauce or dip. Bright, colorful foods may also be more appealing to your child.

283.   Avoid using hydrogenated oils for cooking, and watch out for them in packaged foods. These oils provide no nourishment for your skin or your body. In fact, they actually interfere with "good" oils (olive oil, sunflower oil, flax seed oil, fish oil) ability to nourish your skin, hair, nails and entire body!

284.   Proper nutrition can help you relieve many types of health conditions. Certain types of serious health concerns can be kept under control when you eat

foods that do not make the problem worse. Diabetics can reduce sugar intake and those with high blood pressure can reduce salt and fat.

285.   When trying to have a healthy diet, add new healthy foods. Try something that you have never had before. You may be missing out on something that you really would enjoy. There are a lot of fruits and vegetables that people never try. You can start introducing new foods into your diet slowly. You should try something new once a week.

286.   Make a salad for dinner. You can add chicken, fish, or other lean meats, as well as lots of fresh veggies like carrots, corn, peas, tomatoes and even throw in some strawberries, mandarin oranges or pineapple for some sweet pizazz. Making a salad the entree will keep you from using a high calorie and carbohydrate like pasta instead.

287.   It is important to get enough iron in your diet, because it is used for oxygen transport throughout the body. If you do not get enough, you will suffer from anemia. Good sources of iron include meat, particularly organ meats like liver, dark leafy vegetables such as spinach, and molasses.

288.   Buy fruits and vegetables that are in season. They are widely available, much more flavorful, and

usually less expensive. Try shopping at your local farmer's market, as they will have a great selection. Remember that fruits and vegetables don't last very long. Only buy as much as you know you will eat.

289.   You should try to eat less salty foods to balance out your nutrition and lower sodium levels in your body. By avoiding or eating smaller amounts of foods with high-salt content such as chips, pretzels, pre-packaged noodles, or other foods with large amounts of preservatives, you could receive positive nutritional benefits.

290.   Eat smaller meals every three to four hours. Many people dislike having to stop what they are doing to eat something, so they end up sskipping breakfast, eating lunch late and then overeating at dinner time becuae they are famished. Find mor efficient ways to prepare quick, healthy meals so that you can get the food in your system. This keeps your blood sugar stable, gives you more energy and maintains your mental focus.

291.   Be sure to get enough water in your daily diet. It is vital to a well functioning body and will not only hydrate the skin, it delivers nutrients to the cells and flushes toxins from the body. Many doctors recommend that you drink at least eight glasses of water each day.

292.   To design the most nutritious diet possible, try to only put things into your body that your body can actually use. Fresh fruits, vegetables and meats are best for your body because they are comprised entirely of nutrients that your body can break down and use. Meanwhile, some processed foods and drinks may have low calories or fat, but they also have low nutritional value.

293.   If you want to get a youngster who is a picky-eater to expand his food selection, then try to make a game of it. Experts tell us it can take as many as 10 tries before a child takes easily to a new food you want to introduce. It may work best to provide just one new food at a meal and integrate it with some favorite foods to make it more appealing. Consider cutting new foods up into fun shapes or decorating them with other fun foods you know the child likes. Most importantly, make sure the child sees you eating the food as well. Helping your child get used to new and different foods is a very important part of good nutrition, so trust your instincts, go slow and be patient!

294.   Oprah Winfrey used the phrase "clean eating" in her book Oprah's Kitchen. It's helpful to think of clean eating as a good way to approach food. Simple preparations, lighter salad dressings, using

less oils and fats (though still a bit for flavor!), and keeping things as fresh as possible - all these ideas contribute to her way of clean eating. Oprah loved her fried chicken - and presents a clean way of cooking it in her book. The bottom line is, if you have a choice between fancy and heavy vs. simple and fresh, go with the latter and your scale will thank you, no matter what food you're eating.

295.   Try not to buy into the fact that fruit juices and vegetable juices are a healthy beverage option. Many store bought varieties are riddled with sugar, sodium, and other additives that make them no better than something like a soda. It is best to stick to whole fruits. However, if you do desire fruit juice, the best way is to make your own with a juicer and fresh fruit and vegetables.

296.   Thiamin is an important part of a healthy diet. Thiamin works in the body to help you use energy from carbohydrates effectively. It also helps to regulate your appetite. Muscle function, heart and nervous system are all assisted by this vitamin. Thiamin is found in many foods in small amounts, but you won't find it in refined foods.

297.   If you don't like vegetables, try hiding them in different dishes. For example, vegetable lasagna is usually enjoyed by everyone, even those who don't

enjoy the vegetables. This way, you can get all the really great minerals and vitamins from vegetables without having to eat them in a way that you'd rather not.

298.   Avoid pre-packaged and prepared foods whenever possible if you are looking for the healthiest nutrition. In almost every case pretreated foods and pre-cooked meals feature added ingredients for preservation that are extremely bad for you. It is far better to prepare your own food from fresh ingredients than to rely on food prepared in a factory.

299.   When considering a diet that provides an adequate nutrition level, be sure to include low fat milk. Milk provides many nutrients - including calcium and protein - that the body needs. Studies have shown that drinking milk does benefit both muscle growth, and also the body's ability to maintain a healthy body fat content.

300.   Eat healthful foods to keep your whole body fit and healthy. Your skin will glow if you eat plenty of fresh fruits and veggies, whole grains, proteins, and natural oils. Be sure to get plenty of good oils, such as olive oil, sunflower oil and peanut oil to keep your skin, hair, and nails moisturized, flexible and strong.

301.   Animal fats are seen as culprits of high cholesterol by many nutritionists, so many people are avoiding animal fats. The mainstream recommendation is currently that we make animal fats no more than 10% of our caloric intake. But, there is another voice that says these fats contain necessary nutrients, amino acids that contain carnitine and other substances vital to fat metabolism.

302.   Ginger is a good natural remedy to motion sickness. You can also take ginger in capsule form. Taking 1,000mg of ginger an hour before leaving and for every three hours after that is ideal. Besides preventing an upset stomach, Ginger is known for preventing the nausea caused by travelling. Ginger tea or ginger candy could prove helpful in this situation.

303.   If you are trying to cut down on the amount of soda that you consume and think water is too plain, try flavored water. This tasty alternative comes with the same amount of water that you require, and does not have the high sugar and calorie content as soda.

304.   Make sure that you are getting enough dairy products. Yogurt, eggs. milk, cheese and butter, are

all full of vitamins that our bodies need. The nutrition found in dairy products, cannot be found in any other food group, so it is important that you eat your recommended amount of dairy.

305.   When you are eating out at restaurants, do not add salt to any of your meals. It is common for restaurants to use more salt than you would use at home, so adding more salt to your food will put your food in a very bad sodium range.

306.   Niacin is extremely important to the human body. It forms an integral part of the metabolism in the citric acid cycle, where it serves to help the body turn food into energy. It is found in many meats, seeds, whole grain products and vegetables. Historically, a deficiency of niacin was caused by corn replacing other foods.

307.   Saturated fat consumption is strongly linked to metabolic syndrome, which is the name for the constellation of symptoms that includes, heart disease, high blood pressure, diabetes and high blood cholesterol. In order to reduce your consumption of saturated fat, you should use liquid plant oils, such as olive or peanut oil when possible, for frying, as well as, reducing the consumption of fatty foods in general.

308.   Buy low fat yogurt and make sure you have a bit of it in your fridge. Yogurt is a great meal supplement that is low in calories and fat. It also tastes great and is good for your health. It is also relatively inexpensive, allowing you to keep your food budget low.

www.ingramcontent.com/pod-product-compliance
Lightning Source LLC
Chambersburg PA
CBHW060752260726

48660CB00002B/582